I

HATE

THIS

FEELING

I
HATE
THIS
FEELING

A MEMOIR OF EPILEPSY, BRAIN SURGERY & SEIZURE FREEDOM

JOE RODRIGUEZ

Copyright © 2021 Joseph D. Rodriguez

All rights reserved. No part of this book may be reproduced in any form or by any electronic or mechanical means, including information storage and retrieval systems, without the permission in writing from the author, except by a reviewer who may quote brief passages in a review.

ISBN-13: 978-0-578-87191-2

For me

Table of Contents

PREFACE

What compelled me to write *I Hate This Feeling*?

I had never intended to be a candidate for brain surgery, let alone write a book about my experiences from when I was first diagnosed with epilepsy. However, after reading a memoir titled *Beyond My Control* by Stuart Ross McCallum, I've decided I, too, have a story to tell. I want a written account for me, and anyone interested in my epilepsy journey. If I can help even one person suffering from epilepsy or perhaps help a family member or friend understand what their loved one is going through a little better, that will bring great joy to me.

This book will help readers better understand the process leading up to brain surgery and what can happen afterward. It will also shed light on the type of seizures that I've suffered from - complex partial seizures.

Not too many people know how diverse epilepsy can be. A common misconception is that seizures always exhibit violent shaking and jerking. In my case, those were not the types of seizures that plagued me.

For confidentiality, some names have been changed or left out altogether.

Note: I am not a medical expert. The topics discussed in this book are conveyed to the best of my abilities from memory and notes compiled during my experiences throughout the years. The medical terms I use in this book were presented to me and learned about firsthand from various doctors and relevant medical personnel.

PROLOGUE

It was the night of August 3rd, 2017, and I was standing in my shower around 10 p.m. fighting tears. The warm water, as hot as I could take it, rinsed the tears off my face, the perfect camouflage. These tears were not in vain. I was crying because I was both happy and considerably worried. By the way, it was also my twenty-fourth birthday.

I was in tears because, in a few hours, I would be heading into surgery for an SEEG. This type of EEG would have electrodes implanted into my brain to locate the focus of my epilepsy at last!

Despite the relentless bombardment of worry and the effect the thought of the possibility of the surgery going wrong had had on my psyche the past few months, I was looking forward to the procedure. At this point, with so much time and patience invested in defeating my epilepsy, I was more than ready for the fight.

I was diagnosed with epilepsy in August 2014. August seemed to become a pretty significant month for me - I've met countless doctors and taken countless neurological tests to get to the root of my disorder. Not once did I waver in my pursuit to rectify my biggest health concern.

The proverbial table was set, and all I needed to do was bring the courage and willpower I've maintained over the past several years into the hospital with me on August 4th.

I have always been a sucker for themes in literature, and I cannot help but notice the theme of rebirth. The day after my birthday, I will be admitted into Mount Sinai West in New York City for life-altering surgery. My brain and outlook on life will forever be changed. I will never be who I was before the surgery, and a new part of me will be able to bud, like a flower at the beginning of spring.

If everything goes as planned, I will endure a second surgery days after this, the corrective surgery. Hopefully, these surgeries will free me of this epilepsy and transform me into a person who does not have to worry about being a victim of seizures anymore.

1

IS HEAD TRAUMA TO BLAME FOR MY EPILEPSY?

Aside from the common cold, I was a pretty healthy child growing up in Jersey City, New Jersey. The worst health issue I had as a child happened during the summer of 2001 when I was seven going on eight years old.

During a trip to Bethlehem, Pennsylvania, to visit family, I was at a playground with my two brothers, Lou and D. Lou was twelve at the time while D was four. The day was peaceful while we played as children do. However, I'd encountered a piece of playground equipment I still resent to this very day. This contraption is called a glider. As far as I'm concerned, it's the devil in metal form.

A glider is essentially two vertical metal poles about six feet high, which stand ten to fifteen feet away from each other and are connected at the top by a horizontal beam. Attached to the horizontal beam is a handlebar that slides from one pole to the other. Whenever the handlebar reaches the end of the beam, some type of hydraulic inside slows the handlebar down to make sure the child, who's hanging on for dear life, comes to a "safe" stop. I'm sure I'm not the first person with a glider horror story, and I certainly won't be the last.

The peaceful day turned into a horrible one not long after I had my turn with the glider. I took my grip on the handlebar, and Lou pushed me to the other end. My seven-year-old temperament probably didn't think he pushed me fast enough. That is, until I slammed so forcefully into the other side that I had lost my grip and soared through the air, doing so many backflips I would've impressed the legendary 2016 United States Rio Olympics gymnastics team.

However, the difference between me and the gymnasts is they would've stuck their landing. My landing was hard as I crashed into the wood chips you see at many playgrounds. I can still smell the stench of molding wood emanating from the ground on that hot summer day. Surprisingly my face, hands, and knees weren't covered in splinters from the wood.

The fall knocked every bit of wind right out of me. I

struggled to gain some type of breath, barely able to make it to my feet. Then I hobbled to my grandmother's house nearby.

A trip to the hospital came next where doctors informed me, I had internal bleeding and a ruptured spleen. Surgery was not needed, but I have never felt so much pain in my mid-section since that day and the days following the accident.

Perhaps I should start a petition which will fight to remove every glider from playgrounds in the United States, but I digress.

To this day, my mother, Mabelyn, holds firm that this incident harmed my brain in some way. However, I wasn't concussed. I'm pretty sure there would have been a lot more tests in the hospital than just an ultrasound of my spleen if the doctors felt something wasn't right neurologically. But, hey, mother knows best, right?

Still, knowing why a loved one suffers from a disorder would surely comfort them more than the ailment remaining a mystery. And as much as my mother or anyone else would like to assume the fall may have kickstarted my epilepsy, I remember times when I would get weird, funny feelings when I was only five or six, years

before this playground incident, which only grew worse
as I got older.

2

I'VE GOT A FUNNY FEELING...

At the early age of five or six, I remember feeling like I had superpowers when I would experience moments in real life, which felt like I had dreamed of them before. At that young age, I thought a part of me could tell the future in my dreams. I could be at home playing video games with Lou, and I would get an odd feeling, which would distract me from playing whatever game we were playing at the time.

Back then, at that age, I did not think twice about it. That weird feeling would last ten to fifteen seconds, and then I would move on with my day.

It wasn't until a few years later when my vocabulary grew that I could pair a word with that experience. The word that fits best is déjà vu, which I've always liked when I was younger. The accents above the letters always looked fancy to me, and I enjoyed knowing a fancy word I barely understood.

All I knew was that it described the phenomenon of feeling you've already lived through something. People get déjà vu all the time and feel they are living a moment they have dreamed. Being so young, I'd felt my dreams helped me tell the future.

Of course, I couldn't call upon these dreams at will and predict the future. I would've probably helped my mother win the lottery if that was the case. I knew when I got that déjà vu feeling I had been in that moment in a dream before. It wasn't scary. It was rather intriguing. Déjà vu wasn't a burden, and the brief weird feeling it caused didn't turn me down. It helped me feel like my ability to tell the future was currently activated or turned on.

Just as I was able to understand the term "déjà vu" as I got older and my vocabulary improved, I later ended up learning about a new term in my late teen years: aura.

An aura is a precursor to a seizure. Auras let the person having a seizure know that one is about to strike. Some people with epilepsy, however, don't experience auras, and their seizures sneak attack them. In a way, experiencing auras is both a blessing and a curse. Sure, I'd like to have a warning when a seizure is about to happen, but the way the auras made me feel as I got older made me wish I had never experienced them at all.

I will use the term aura to refer to the physiological phenomenon, which occurred before my seizures from here on out, even for the times I describe before my diagnosis and before I knew what auras were.

3

GLEEFUL TO DEFLATED

During my high school years, I was a bit overweight. But I was healthy enough to make my high school's varsity baseball team as a freshman and play all four years. It was a great time for me. The small charter school I had attended was a microcosm of the city where we all grew up. It was rich in diversity and operated by a staff that cared about their students. I wasn't popular by any means, but the combination of my being on the baseball team and the small school population meant I was pretty sociable and knew almost everyone in my grade level.

Some classes were better than others. One of the better classes was called study hall, an elective that mainly upper-level students took when it was clear we had enough credit hours to graduate.

We were supposed to study, but that did not always

happen. There were times when students, including me, took a reprieve from the rigors of the school day and relaxed and socialized.

The study hall I had taken my senior year of high school was a special one because it took place at the end of the day, twice a week. My friends and I relished in the fact that for us, school pretty much ended after the period before study hall on those days. The glee I'd felt when I was in that class was great. There was one day in particular, though, I remember getting an aura, which felt unlike any that came before.

At the time, I had no idea I was having a seizure. I remember having a pretty good time in class just having conversations, and then I felt something creeping up on me. My friends, unaware of anything happening to me internally, carried on none the wiser. As it crept closer, I became worried. The funny feeling that came and went throughout my childhood seemed to have evolved. Something which used to not even be intrusive in the slightest became a behemoth. It made my thoughts swirl around like my brain was in a blender.

There was also a feeling of gloom that came over me. It originated from somewhere in my torso and radiated outward. My arms, hands, legs, and feet all felt disconnected from my body. In all, it lasted anywhere from forty-five to sixty seconds, but it felt like an eternity. This first of many crippling auras made me feel like I was in utter despair. I would say this feeling is exponentially worse than any panic or anxiety attack.

My seventeen-year-old self was ignorant when it came to epilepsy and seizures. I was a layman like many people are when it comes to epilepsy. I'd thought this was a freak incidence of random dizziness. I was happy to be sitting down.

During the time it took the aura to grip me and let me go, I did not care about anything except myself. I withdrew from whatever conversation was going on, and I guess I kept up a good enough façade to keep them from catching onto the crisis I had endured.

During the aura, I felt like I wasn't even a part of the group anymore. I was detached from reality like life was going on without me. When I tell you that my auras are probably one of the worst things one could ever physically experience, I mean it.

There's a scene in one of my favorite movies, which somewhat depicts my inner crisis rather fittingly. Those of you who aren't nerds and haven't seen *The Lord of the Rings: The Fellowship of the Ring*, allow me to set the scene for you.

The point of the movie is for the lead character, Frodo, to destroy a powerful ring by throwing it into the fiery depths of a volcano. The journey won't be easy, so various warriors were chosen to help escort Frodo to the volcano. During their meeting, an argument erupts, and all hell breaks loose. Despite the arguing, Frodo is gripped by the ring's power, which speaks to him and holds his attention. No one notices Frodo's despair, and he is utterly uninterested in all the arguing going on since all he can think about is this ring's powerful grip on him.

I've had seizures in public, and much like Frodo, the seizures gripped me to the point where nothing else in the moment mattered. I've been in busy locations where there's a lot of hustle and bustle, and once a seizure starts, everything going on around me dissolves. The cars driving by and the people rushing past me don't notice my despair, and I'm equally not worried about them. The aura takes my full attention, and the resulting seizure completely alters my consciousness but more on that later.

Being able to feel a seizure approach gives you a heads up to get ready but in return makes you feel like complete crap. Also, knowing I should get away from a crowd when I would feel an aura coming was good but couldn't always be accomplished.

Still, I did well in high school, graduating in 2011 with the third-highest GPA in a class of over one hundred students.

4

COLLEGE

I had attended Rutgers University in Newark, New Jersey, from 2011 to 2016. I only lived on campus during my first year. It was fun, but it wasn't for me. Plus, my home was close enough to the school to make commuting tolerable, so living on campus wasn't completely justifiable.

Classes were good, and I was happy to be on my way to a degree. However, sometimes I would think back to the auras I would get in high school and worry about them.

Strangely, my auras increased while I was living on campus. I'd spent many nights staying up late, completing assignments, and watching movies on Netflix. There was something peaceful about being up all night and being awake to see daylight creep into my tiny two-bed dorm room.

On many occasions where I pulled all-nighters, I'd, of course, be groggy to start the next day, but at some point, I'd get an aura, especially if I did not get a full night's sleep. I think it'd be safe to say the uptick in auras I'd experience after an all-nighter should have led me to knock it off and get more sleep.

The following year, I worried about these weird feelings becoming more frequent, but I didn't make the connection between my lack of sleep and the auras. I knew I was getting these "dizzy feelings" more frequently. So, I looked into some neurologists in my area with the hope they'd be able to tell me what was going on.

I ended up finding a doctor who was in-network with my insurance and located close by in a neighboring city. I won't give away his location or name, however, because I don't have much good to say about him now that I know what was happening to me and due to his lack of initiative, which made him not look more carefully into my concerns.

When I had met this doctor, he struck me as being very quirky. After a few minutes, I knew he wasn't the guy for me. He went through the motions and asked me what problems I was experiencing. I told him I would feel dizzy and like my world was spinning, which would result in me feeling depleted.

He followed up by taking my pulse and listening to my heartbeat. Then he followed it up by doing an eye test where I tracked his pen by not moving my head. Finally, I had to walk toward and away from him, one foot in front of the other, toe to heel. That was pretty much the entire visit. His diagnosis?

Stress.

He recommended I stress less. Neither MRIs nor EEGs were conducted. There wasn't even blood work done! During the ride home, I was just as confused about my condition as when I walked into the doctor's office. I knew a lot of college students, at the time, who were as stressed as I was, and not one of them ever complained about getting dizzy spells. My mother commented on how odd the doctor was. I couldn't disagree. He was strange. Maybe this guy stole the real doctor's white coat and filled in for him for the day, and I never actually got to see the real doctor.

With the diagnosis of stress and me being a layman, I decided to take the doctor's advice and try to stress less. That didn't do much because I continued to get these weird feelings. However, I tried to ignore them because like the doctor said, it was just stress, right?

To reduce my "attacks," he suggested I start taking better care of myself, so I diligently started eating better and exercising.

Over the next few months, my weight dropped from 205 pounds to 165 pounds. I gave up drinking soda and haven't had any since. That was quite an accomplishment because having sugary, caffeinated beverages was always great, but it got me thinking. Perhaps it was a reason I had seizures.

If the auras stopped as a result of my healthier eating, then my poor diet must have been the cause of my seizures all along. There's nothing worse in the world than thinking you are sabotaging your body, and that alone was enough stress for me to try to shoulder!

There was a time I'd felt Oreos caused my seizures. I know it seems silly, but when you're at your wit's end, you'll do anything you can to find out what you can do to stop your dreaded seizures.

I may have lost forty pounds, but it did nothing for my seizure disorder. My episodes didn't slow down and, oddly enough, may have picked up as time passed.

Although my studies continued in a positive direction, I felt I was all alone in my battle with epilepsy, and while I wouldn't say I became depressed, I wasn't always feeling my best. There was not much I felt like I could do to ease the state of angst the fear of seizures always had me in.

Some things I've done might not have been much help, like smoking cigarettes. There was no gateway to introduce me to it. One day, while feeling downtrodden due to my seizures, I bought a pack of Marlboro Silvers, and that was that. I kept it a secret. At first, I felt weird smoking outside. Even though no one cared about some guy smoking, I felt like everyone was judging me. I knew my family would not understand, and I tried to keep it hidden from them. I made sure to do it in the backyard if I was at home when no one else was outside.

There was something peaceful about it, especially at night when it was nice and cool with a slight drizzle. Those smoking sessions were quite relaxing. I don't want to romanticize smoking, however. I knew it wasn't good for me, but with all the added stress about never knowing when my next seizure would hit, I took joy in the peaceful moments I could get.

5

AUTOPILOT

As the years passed, my auras did not get any better. I guessed that I was just a stressed individual. I had stopped seeing my neurologist and did not seek help anywhere else. However, it may have behooved me to get a second opinion.

I credit my younger brother, D, for noticing something very odd about my actions following my aura phase. He tried to convince me that a blank stare would develop on my face and I would smack my lips constantly, but I never believed him. I just fired back at him that I would know if I was doing such weird things. I dismissed the observations as being silly because I knew I wasn't doing that. I'm myself after all, and I felt I had a pretty good idea about what was going on with my body.

However, he never relented. Whenever I was

around him, or anyone I trusted, I'd murmur that I was getting dizzy. If I were with D, he'd most likely wait until I got through the aura to let me know about his observations. And I'd still constantly deny his claims.

This situation and my dilemma continued for the next couple of years. My auras were increasing, but I would weather the storm every time. I still had no idea these feelings were seizures. However, there was one eye-opening moment for me.

It occurred in January 2014 during the second semester of my third year of college. I no longer lived on campus and easily commuted from Jersey City to Newark.

I was heading to the Journal Square Transportation Center where there is a bus terminal as well as the PATH train system. The PATH trains can get you to New York City or Newark in minutes. I took the Newark train to get to Rutgers every morning.

My walk to the terminal started as it usually did, tedious and boring. During the walk, I began to get an aura. I felt the usual sense of panic and impending doom. Then, before I knew it, I was standing at an intersection, muttering random things to a man standing to my right.

"I hate this feeling," I said.

"Excuse me? Are you okay?" The man's eyes were almost bulging out of his head.

He seemed genuinely concerned about me. He must've been wondering who I was, why I was muttering things to him, and if I should be getting help from proper medical personnel.

I told him, "Yes. . . yes, I'm okay. Thank you."

Once again, I weathered the storm. However, this time, things were different. This time I had realized something eye-opening. I did not recall seeing the man before my aura. I also did not recall the events, which led me to end up standing next to him.

I realized I must have blacked out.

Shortly after my aura started, it was as if my body went into autopilot. The lights were on, but nobody was home. I was unconscious but still able to walk and maneuver normally. Something made me stop at the beginning of the intersection and talk to that man. The event replays in my head even though I do not recall any of it. I always wonder: *What if that man hadn't been there? Would I have just kept walking into traffic and gotten killed?*

We were waiting at the intersection for a reason.

The light was green. Cars were zooming past us at this busy intersection. Had the man not been there, I may have walked right into traffic. The thought of that makes me shudder.

Although I wasn't consciously present, some part of me knew I had to stop and wait at the intersection. I do not know why my mind decided talking to the man was a good idea, though.

At the end of my commute and before my class, I called Lou to let him know about what had happened. He's probably the most facetious person I know. He'll take any serious topic and try to make a joke about it. But maybe it's less about him being uncouth and more about him trying to make the tough moments easier to handle for all of us.

I vaguely recall the discussion we had over the phone. My mind was still racing from the events I had just endured. However, I recall Lou making some sort of joke about what the man I was muttering to must've been thinking.

Despite the uneasiness I was feeling, I still went to class. Auras knew no bounds. I got them in several classes as their frequency increased. Still, I figured anyone in college was stressing as much as I was, if not more. At that time, I didn't do anything to combat the stress. I went with the flow for lack of a better explanation.

My uneasiness increased after I had an aura during one of my classes in a lecture hall, and it provided an unbiased opinion.

So, there I was in a lecture hall, the worst place to feel the panic of an aura and impending seizure coming. Like many times before, I knew what was up and just wanted to get away from everyone. However, I stayed in my seat. Big mistake or maybe not!

When I came to, a classmate I was friendly with at the time looked concerned. He said in a low voice as to not interrupt the science lesson, "Bro, it looked like you were on something!" He was referring to my blank stare and lip-smacking.

I never gave him a heads up that I was about to have a seizure, nor did he know about my condition. It wasn't like D had a conversation with him and told him to look out for lip-smacking. He noticed on his own. Although auras made me feel like utter crap when they came, they gave me notice of what was about to happen. I'd hoped there'd be a time I'd be able to use that bit of knowledge to get away and not have to endure the embarrassment of having seizures in front of people.

During my college political science class, I had another mid-class seizure. I felt the aura sneaking up on me and had just enough warning to drag myself out of my seat and into the hallway until my seizure subsided. Luckily, that one instance, I was able to get away from the crowd by leaving class and seeking refuge in the hallway, but I knew I wouldn't always be so lucky in the future.

There was also a time in 2014 when I worked as a cashier in one of the largest liquor stores in New Jersey. It gets massive foot traffic with long lines, and there was a time I was checking out a young couple's items when I had felt an aura starting.

Although my first instinct was to get away and hide, the fear always crippled me, and I tried to continue my work. Before I knew it, a coworker was beside me finishing the transaction, and the couple I was initially helping was very concerned.

The couple as well as my coworker kept asking me if I was okay. I assured them I was and thanked them, and then I went back to work like nothing happened because that's all I knew. It was what I did.

I wouldn't say time slowed down during my auras, but at the onset of an aura, a feeling of great angst took hold of me. Talk about stress! But I just went on with living, went on with working and with school.

Since I had little luck with my first neurologist, I figured things would be what they were, but I felt I had to seek out a second opinion if I wanted an actual chance to get some answers.

6

NEW DOCTOR

With my mother's help, I found a new neurologist nearby. She seemed nice. She was an older woman, so I knew she had been doing this for a long time. With all that experience, I was hoping she'd be the one to help me.

My first appointment with her consisted of me letting her know all about my symptoms. "I get a weird feeling that starts somewhere in my mid-section. Then it seems to radiate to the rest of my body. It makes me feel uncomfortable," I said. I also mentioned how my brother tells me post-episode that I smack my lips and mumble, but I have no recollection of it.

Just like my neurologist from a couple of years ago, she conducted some simple tests on me. She read my heart rate, checked my breathing, made me follow her finger without moving my head, and checked my reflexes. Based on my description of my symptoms, she deduced it was a form of epilepsy called petit mal seizures. Petit mal seizures are a general term for seizures where the affected person exhibits the symptoms of a brief loss of consciousness.

Although the person is not unconscious in the literal sense of sleeping, they are unaware of anything that's going on and appear to be awake.

She also explained that the weird feeling I was experiencing was called an aura. "Auras occur before a seizure takes place. Not all people who suffer from seizures have auras, but for those who do, auras kind of act like a warning that one is about to take place," she said.

Another way to describe this affliction is called absence seizures. Although my diagnosis seemed like an educated guess based on my description of my symptoms, I felt like I was finally getting somewhere.

The doctor ordered an EEG, which measures electrical activity in the brain. Then, if I was lucky, the doctor could confirm a general area where the seizures were originating. She also prescribed me a medication called ethosuximide, an anti-convulsant medication, with a dosage of 250 mg two times a day.

What was once a mystery for so many years was finally brought out into the light.

I had epilepsy.

I was an epileptic.

I suffered from recurrent seizures.

Those funny feelings I had before I was ten years old were auras. I was having seizures when all I thought was happening were simple déjà vu events, which were followed by dizziness.

Despite the news that I was an epileptic, I was glad I had a doctor who was no-nonsense and figured something out. She didn't give me the run around, and she didn't belittle my symptoms and insist they were stress related. She knew what she was doing and had a plan for me. If an EEG is what she wanted me to get, then I would get an EEG.

7

FIRST EEG

Since I was a psychology major at Rutgers University, I had some background knowledge about EEGs. I knew they didn't hurt, and I also knew the worst part about them would be slight itchiness from the gel residue left over on the scalp after the test is complete. So, with that knowledge, I was ready to see how the experience would play out.

I had my EEG scheduled at Hoboken University Medical Center in Hoboken, New Jersey, and I got checked in quickly. The entire process leading up to the start of the EEG was downright pleasant.

I removed my glasses as the EEG tech prepped their station. I had to sit straight up for the application of the electrodes. During an EEG, about a dozen electrodes attached to a computer by wire are strategically placed all over the scalp for the EEG to be able to read individual parts of the brain simultaneously.

After I got comfortable, the EEG tech went to work. Before applying a gel, which holds the electrodes in place and assists the computer in reading my brain activity, they gently scrubbed the part of my scalp where they had to attach the electrodes. The gentle scrubbing was quite relaxing, and I found myself enjoying the process of electrode application.

It was so relaxing that I lost track of time, but after about ten minutes, I was told to lie down. The tech told me that there would be two parts to the test. The first part required me to close my eyes while they set up a lighting fixture above my face, which would rapidly flash different colored lights. The idea is that flashing lights can trigger seizures in certain individuals, and if my electrical brain activity got disrupted in the slightest, the EEG would pick it up.

The second part was what I found to be the least enjoyable. I had to hyperventilate for five minutes straight, which could also induce seizures in certain individuals and, at the least, have an effect on my brain, which could tell my doctor where my seizures were coming from.

The light test was a piece of cake. Although the flashing lights can get quite annoying, all you're doing is lying still and letting the machine do the work. The hyperventilation portion highly juxtaposes the light portion of the test. The EEG tech let me know that once I started to hyperventilate, I could not stop until he told me to. With that bit of info, I was ready to start.

Quick, rapid breaths rushed in and out of my mouth. It wasn't long until I felt a slight tingling sensation in my head, which made me feel extremely uncomfortable. The tingling migrated to my lips and then to my extremities. I thought: *I have to do THIS for five minutes straight?*

As the minutes passed, my body began to squirm out of exhaustion and discomfort. The tech let me know where I was on the timer.

"Three minutes left."

The physiological response the hyperventilating caused was so uncomfortable. I honestly hated the tingles, which developed all over my body. It was hard for me to stay still. Also, for some reason, I felt like my face and lips were getting pale while hyperventilating, and that made me uneasy as well. Nevertheless, I knew I had to persevere for the test to be as accurate as possible and provide the answers I was looking for.

"Two minutes left."

I struggled to stay aware of my surroundings, feeling nauseous and dizzy.

"One minute left."

Getting close, I knew I had to hang on just a bit longer.

"Three, two, one. Okay, breathe normally now."

I was met with instant relief the moment I was able to slow down my breathing. I couldn't see my face, but I'm sure my lips were pale. Neither the light test nor the hyperventilating induced a seizure, but I was hoping the combination would be enough to show my doctor what she needed to find out what was going on.

The electrodes were then unceremoniously removed. They yanked them off with one swift tug. Surprisingly, it wasn't as enjoyable as the application.

The EEG tech used a damp cloth to scrub my head to remove the gel residue. After they finished, I still felt some gel on my scalp, so I asked if I could scrub it myself until I felt it was nice and clean.

The EEG was complete! My instructions were to

follow up with my doctor in a few days so we could discuss the results and see what our next steps would be.

39

8

NORMAL

The follow-up visit with my doctor was not long after my EEG. I was eager to find out what the results
were naturally. After waiting anxiously in the doctor's
office, I finally got called in to hear the news, which
wasn't good, but it wasn't bad either. It was puzzling.

My EEG results came back normal, no abnormal
electrical activity in my brain. I honestly wished there
was something to find so we could put our finger on the
problem and work toward a solution. The doctor explained that normal readings could happen despite a person having epilepsy. Sometimes, the only way to find
seizure activity during an EEG is actually to have a seizure during it. In my case, having a seizure during the
EEG would've been a big help.

I lived every day hoping not to have a seizure, but
during an EEG would've been the one time I would

have welcomed it. It seems quite contradictory to have that logic, but I was desperate for answers.

My doctor suggested an MRI, which uses powerful magnets to get a glimpse at organs in the body, in this case, the brain. They are often used for athletes to ascertain whether or not they may have muscle injuries. The MRI would show my doctor detailed images of my brain and allow her to see if there were any brain lesions. Brain lesions result from past head trauma and are visible on MRI imaging. If that horrific fall at the playground many years ago did hurt my brain, the doctor would see damage in some part of it.

I was all for it. Once again, like EEGs, my psychology education already taught me about MRIs. I knew they were pretty simple. Although I'd have to lie on my back like during the EEG, I would have to do no work. There would be no flashing lights or hyperventilating to make me uncomfortable.

For a lot of people who get MRIs of the brain, the biggest hurdle is the feeling of claustrophobia from the imaging device.

To begin with, you get to wear a skimpy little gown and lie on a thin gurney-like platform that slowly pulls you into the center of this large doughnut looking con-traption. The being in the middle of this is what can mess with people's psyche and cause them to quit the test. I was never a claustrophobic person, so I wasn't too worried. That part would be easy.

9

MRI

Like my EEG appointment, my MRI was scheduled in Hoboken. It took place in a small, unassuming office near the waterfront that overlooks the New York City skyline. Again, the experience was quite pleasant. I know that sounds weird.

After entering the MRI offices, I was told to remove anything magnetic from my person. My mother came with me for this appointment, so I gave her my glasses, belt, wallet and necklace. Leaving something like a credit card on your person can result in it being rendered unusable. The strong magnets of the MRI can erase the magnetic stripe of credit and debit cards. So, out they go while the MRI is in use.

The machine was quite large and took up most of the room. I was given instructions not to move at all during the test. As I lay down on the cold white surface, the technician handed me a button like those used on a game show to buzz in when you know the correct answer. That's not what it was meant for.

Instead, my button was in case I was claustrophobic and started to panic. A simple squeeze would halt the test and send me squeaking back out from inside the middle of the doughnut.

I made sure I understood all the instructions and was ready for my test to commence. However, the formalities were not over. They gave me a packet of earplugs because the machine could be quite loud, and it'd be in my best interest to make sure they were in my ears snuggly.

I opened the packet and smushed a plug into each ear. Finally, I lay down but still needed final preparation. The MRI technician centered me the best he could on the table, and with my head inside a circular apparatus protruding from the gurney, he placed bits of foam blocks between my head and the apparatus to close the gaps, which would keep my head from moving.

After my head was secured, the tech left the test room for the control room. I was slowly pushed into the doughnut. I lay there patiently knowing the test would shortly be underway, but suddenly, the most annoying thing happened. My nose started to itch! I quickly scratched before the test started but to no avail. The itch was relentless. It's funny how things work out this way. It was as if my body was playing a prank on me. I knew I needed to remain still, which meant I would have to put mind over matter and power through. The EEG caused discomfort by hyperventilation while the MRI caused discomfort by itch. Who would've ever thought I'd encounter that dilemma?

After I got my last scratch out of the way, the test commenced. As the MRI started to do its work, I understood why I needed earplugs. The MRI made many different sounds. In the beginning, there was a sound akin to the sound of a train rolling along tracks – *chugga, chugga,* but without any horns or whistles that would accompany a train.

Then there were very loud, rapid, zap sounds that could be likened to a blaster gun out of a Star Wars movie. These were extremely loud. I'm glad I was wearing earplugs. The sounds droned on, became monotonous, and then suddenly stopped. However, before long, they started up again to catch you by surprise. Oddly enough, as I lay there, I was actually able to doze off despite the sounds, which was beneficial because MRIs can be quite long - anywhere from thirty minutes to an hour. If I fell asleep, the test would appear to fly by, I wouldn't need to hear the loud sounds, and the itch, which still bugged me, wouldn't be such a nuisance.

The MRI finished up, and the tech made the machine pull the gurney out from the center of the doughnut. I was glad it was over. Despite me thinking it wouldn't be as bad as the EEG, it wasn't as relaxing as I thought it'd be. However, I never felt claustrophobic. My itchy nose was the worst part. So, what I'm trying to say is, MRIs aren't bad at all.

After I got back to the waiting room, I met my mother, who gave me my belongings. I was promised a disc so I could have it for my records and review it at home. I thought that was pretty cool. The disc had my name written on it along with the office's name.

I was very eager to view it for myself. When I got home, I inserted the disc into my computer and feasted my eyes upon my brain! I was able to look at individual layers or slices of my brain to see each part of it individually. I'd realized this would help the doctor get an in-depth look, so she'd be able to detect if any possible lesions were present.

I couldn't wait for my next doctor's visit so I could get her expert opinion.

However, that eagerness quickly turned sour once I found out the MRI read as normal. There was no evidence of brain trauma or lesions. My doctor explained that these things happen with some epilepsy patients.

If there was a stage before square one, that's where I was. I had no answers and was still having seizures. The feeling I had was like walking in a dark tunnel with no flashlight or idea how to escape. I was trapped. My medication wasn't helping, but the doctor insisted I stay on it with the hope that things would turn around for the better.

10

REPORTED

In the summer of 2014, there was a disheartening time when the auras wore me to a point where I couldn't cope with them anymore. Each one seemed to take a little more out of me. The start of an aura was like a punch to my gut from a heavyweight boxer. Then the way my mind swirled after the aura was over was like I got punched in the head right after.

I suppose my mother was at her wit's end because she took me to a local ER after I complained about getting an aura one day. This trip was like no other.

I described my symptoms to the woman at the ER desk, and she took my info and asked me to have a seat. I waited and waited and finally met a nurse who took me to a bed. Then, once again, I explained my symptoms to her.

"I get a weird feeling throughout my body that makes me feel uncomfortable. The feeling goes all over my body, and I end up feeling worn out and exhausted," I said.

My mother described the lip-smacking and blank stare that my younger brother always mentioned as well, which was a key piece of information.

The nurse continued taking notes. She asked me if I had ever wet myself during these episodes before.

Wet myself? Could that actually happen?

"No. Never," I replied.

I couldn't fathom the embarrassment and hopelessness I'd feel if after an aura was over, I looked down to discover I'd urinated myself. I never wanted to be in that predicament, and the fact the nurse made a point to ask me that question put that possibility in my head and terrified me.

Not long after the questioning was over, the doctor on staff rushed in and barely introduced herself. I don't even recall her name, but she had a big impact on my life. She demanded my driver's license. She explained that I was having seizures, which I already knew.

It was explained to me a person who suffers from

seizures could not operate a vehicle under any circumstances. Although I did not own a car and did not drive at all, my mother was far too scared to ever let me drive her car even before she knew I was having seizures; the doctor still needed to report me.

She input my driver's license number into some database and handed it back to me. I wasn't sure what would happen next. I assumed I'd receive some letter in the mail letting me know about what the doctor had done.

I wasn't in the ER for long. I was discharged with instructions to follow up with my neurologist about the visit. All I could think was, *my license will be gone, and I still have no answers.* I felt hopeless.

11

SUSPENDED

It wasn't long before I received a letter in the mail on behalf of the New Jersey Department of Motor Vehicles, which requested I fill out a form that would list pertinent information regarding my epilepsy. I would have to note my last three recent seizures, if they occurred while I was awake or asleep as well as what medications I was on at the time. I had recently started taking another medication called Keppra, which was also supposed to help my seizure frequency.

There was also a portion for my neurologist to fill out. This section had questions for her with the big one found at the bottom of the page. The final question asked my neurologist if she thought I was fit to operate a motor vehicle despite my epilepsy. To my surprise, she noted that I was fit to operate one. Although I was having recurring seizures, she thought I should be eligible to drive.

In hindsight, it might not have been the right decision since my seizures continued. Still, it made me feel somewhat better about the situation. She might not have wanted to jump the gun and suspend me because we were still pretty new to each other, and I may have, with time, had a chance to get some control over my epilepsy.

My neurologist's faith in me was all for naught. Not long after mailing my response letter to the DMV, they sent me their verdict. The letter, dated July 10th, 2014, read:

Your New Jersey driving privilege is scheduled to be suspended as of 08/09/2014 indefinitely. The Motor Vehicle Commission has information indicating that you are not medically and/or physically able to operate a motor vehicle safely because you are subject to seizures.

Reading this was like a punch to the gut. For some reason, I thought my doctor's belief in me would sway their decision. However, that was not the case. A person with epilepsy cannot drive if they've had a seizure within the past six months. I had had three within a few weeks. The motor vehicle commission saw the number of seizures I had and probably stopped right there. My doctor's opinion meant nothing when I had that many seizures so recently.

My license status wasn't the only change to happen. Another change happened as well, a big one. Not long after my driver's license got suspended, my neurologist let me know she was retiring, and I'd have to find someone new. I wasn't sure what to make of this. I had lost my privilege to drive and now my doctor, who struck me as someone who was trying hard to help me.

And it meant I would have to start from scratch again with a new doctor. That meant introducing myself as well as recounting my symptoms and starting a new relationship, which may or may not work. At the time, I would've bet on the latter based on how defeated I felt. However, this new doctor turned out to become a beacon of hope for me.

12

A NEW BEGINNING

Starting over is never fun, and that's what I felt was happening when I had first met Dr. Kapoor in 2015. However, I was pleasantly surprised, and I'm comfortable using his name because he was such a professional and caring doctor. Talking to him during our appointments felt like talking to a friend. A quote I'll always remember from our first meeting was, "We will get your license back."

Dr. Kapoor was the catalyst for everything good that happened to me regarding beating my epilepsy. When I'd first met him, he immediately seemed like someone I could hang out with. He was young and seemed down to earth. There were many neurological tests I would have and people whom I would later meet through him, which ultimately helped me.

After a few visits, I was very comfortable with Dr. Kapoor. He started my treatment by researching all of the tests and background from my previous retired neurologist, and he got right to work, sending me to whom he thought would be able to help me next. I also had some intriguing videos to show him as well.

There were a couple of occasions where I've used the warnings my auras gave me to my advantage. After feeling the onset of an aura, I was able to take out my phone and quickly navigate to the camera and put it on selfie mode. Amazingly, I was able to record myself having a seizure and see for myself what transpired. D was right all along! I was able to see the lip-smacking and hear the gibberish I mumbled. I'm not sure how I was able to keep the camera aimed at my face, but luckily, I was successful.

I still have those two videos, and I don't show them to anyone. They make me shudder. However, it was smart on my part. Showing those videos to Dr. Kapoor helped him get a good idea of what was afflicting me before ever having seizures with EEG equipment attached to me. These videos said a thousand words, more than just recounting my symptoms ever could.

Dr. Kapoor was intrigued by these videos and referred me to a doctor who specialized in epilepsy, an epileptologist, whose office was nearby and could evaluate me further.

Epileptologists are experts in epileptic seizures and are sometimes the last hope when other treatments intended to stop seizures have failed. This doctor, whom I do not want to name, met with me, and I once again recounted all of my symptoms. Recounting your symptoms, especially when they're as challenging to describe as auras are, becomes taxing after a while.

In mid-2015, I was scheduled for a video EEG by Dr. Kapoor, and the new epileptologist. A video EEG is similar to a regular EEG concerning the electrode and application process. However, you must be admitted to the hospital where you'll be receiving it since you'll be there for several days. The objective is to induce a seizure while in the hospital, hopefully.

The video part comes in because there is a monitor beside your bed with a camera attached. The camera is always recording, so you want to make sure you are cognizant of that and not end up picking your nose or doing anything else weird. However, if you have a seizure, it'll record what kind of actions you display while a seizure is occurring. You also have a small purse-like bag with straps to keep the EEG hardware on your body in case you have to get up to stretch or go to the bathroom.

The "purse" houses electronics that use the electrodes on the scalp to read brain activity and relay it to the nearby computer. There is also a button that notes the exact time you have a seizure if pressed in time. It'll allow the epileptologist to jump right to an event if one happens. Luckily, since I've experienced auras before my seizures, the button would come in handy since I'd have the wherewithal to press it.

I had the normal EEG electrodes applied to my scalp, was hooked up to the "purse" and given my button.

Each day, my epileptologist observed the brain activity and came to speak with me, perhaps to lift my spirits, because I felt like I could tap out at any moment. I was stir-crazy and hadn't showered in days. After the third day and no seizures, I tapped out. I felt like I had wasted my time since I still had no answers. However, a part of me hoped the lengthy EEG would give them a little info regarding why I had seizures.

Dr. Kapoor said the findings were pretty lackluster, and I'd have to go back for another video EEG. I was feeling really dejected, but the doctors suggested a different approach for my next video EEG. This time, my epileptologist stopped all my medications, and I sleep deprived myself. Without taking my medications regularly, a withdrawal effect should occur, which would induce seizures. Sleep deprivation would also elicit seizures as well. I couldn't help but think about all the all-nighters I'd pulled in college and realized they were causing those seizures back then when I thought they were just dizzy spells.

This time, we had more success. In fact, I had a seizure on my first night. When I felt the aura, I clicked that button to let my epileptologist know exactly where to look for a change in brain activity. However, I didn't stop at one seizure. I needed to have one or two more to confirm the seizure I had and the location it occurred in wasn't an isolated incident.

So, I stayed off my meds and refused to sleep, and I had two more seizures. My epileptologist seemed more optimistic during visits to my room, and my stay was shorter than my previous one.

Dr. Kapoor received all the information from the epileptologist, and I was scheduled for another test to further verify the findings. Positron emission tomography (PET) is another way to get a look at the brain, much like an MRI. The PET scan is conducted like an MRI with regard to there being a doughnut instrument to lie inside, but there is an injection involved, which administers a tracer, which reacts with the machine in order to better assess the body part in question. The injection was no big deal, and neither was the lying still. However, I may have gotten a nose itch during the process. How great? The test was completed without an issue, and I had to wait for my results.

The description of the findings read:

Asymmetrical decreased metabolic activity of the right temporal/hippocampal lobe. This suggests that the seizure focus is on the right.

This data was invaluable. During my next appointment with Dr. Kapoor, he explained to me what all the data we now had suggested. My seizures were coming from my right temporal lobe. The temporal lobes involve speech and memory. The location of my seizure activity may have been why I blacked out during my seizures and muttered things. He diagnosed me with complex partial seizures.[1] During complex partial seizures, the person afflicted will lose awareness and often exhibit automatisms. Automatisms were explained to me as actions that are performed without conscious awareness. The lip-smacking and gibberish rambling exhibited my automatisms. There was more testing to do.

Over several months, I had more neuropsychological testing done. After several tests, my epileptologist suggested a fairly invasive procedure that included brain mapping to locate the exact seizure focus as well as the possible removal of my entire right temporal lobe. I never saw him again.

Instead, I returned to Dr. Kapoor, who never jumped to such rash decisions.

---

[1] According to Epilepsy.com, complex partial seizures have been renamed and are now called focal impaired awareness seizures. I will continue to call them complex partial seizures in this writing, because that is how I knew them at the time.

13

OVERDOSE

My seizure frequency hadn't changed, but what did change were my medications. Dr. Kapoor took me off of one of my first epilepsy medications, ethosuximide, and paired Keppra with a newer, more promising drug called Vimpat.

I'd felt Keppra always gave me a bad mood and no relief from my seizures and a constant reminder of serious side effects based on the label affixed to the bottle, which read, "May cause suicidal ideations." This was less than ideal.

As it turned out, Keppra, along with Vimpat, combined to nearly take me under.

During the summer of 2015, I was on 1500 mg of Keppra twice a day and 200 mg of Vimpat twice a day. I took the Keppra in 500 mg pills, so I had to take three pills for each 1500 mg dose. One night, I was supposed to go out to watch *Avengers: Age of Ultron* with an old friend who came by to pick me up.

We figured we would be out late and thought I could be late for my nighttime dose, so I decided to take it before I left for the movie. My room was a bit dark, but I felt I could still make out the bottles based on feel.

I was supposed to take three 500 mg Keppra pills and one 200 mg Vimpat pill. However, I took one Vimpat pill, put the bottle down, and then accidentally picked it back up and took three more. Big mistake.

I didn't notice anything out of the ordinary until I got to my friend's car and started to feel my heart beating harder and faster than normal. My vision got blurry, and my lips began to tingle. Uh, oh.

I told my friend what was going on and apologized. My mother's boyfriend, Hector, was home at the time, and I called to let him know what was going on. He offered to drive me to Hoboken University Medical Center's ER. I apologized to my friend and got out of the car to walk the ten steps back home.

Hector drove me to the hospital where I was admitted very quickly. A big concern for the doctors was if I ever had any suicidal thoughts, and they asked me that explicitly. I told them no, this was an honest mistake. I was given fluids and kept in the ER for a couple of hours but was discharged not too long after around 9 p.m. once the side effects subsided.

My mother worked at a doctor's office, just a block from the hospital at the time, and was able to get there immediately. I was very worried about all the physiological responses going on with my body, and seeing her worry made me more scared. Luckily, it wasn't a life-threatening overdose. To this day, I still haven't watched that Avengers movie.

14

A REGULAR LIFE

For most people, normal is boring. It's no different when you are battling epilepsy, but most of us would take boring for a while if it meant feeling normal in the usual clinical sense. I did my best, but having seizures put a damper on things.

For the past couple of years, I'd thought about nothing but college and my seizure activity. However, after graduating from college in May 2016, I had some room to enjoy some of the simpler things in life. My Yankees fandom never wavered over the years, and I had a thought about getting a tattoo. Perhaps, this stemmed from never having much control over a lot of things. A tattoo would be done on my terms and thus make it under my control.

I enjoyed pondering what kind of a tattoo to get. It seemed like the possibilities were endless. However, I knew I wanted something to signify my epilepsy battle, but I couldn't figure out how I wanted it to be executed.

I thought about getting a purple ribbon since purple signifies epilepsy, and a purple ribbon is a sign of epilepsy awareness. However, I didn't feel like that was creative enough. Then I stumbled on the geometric tattoo design style while looking at tattoo design ideas and wondered what a geometric brain would look like.

It was at the same time that I had decided a minimalist tattoo would speak more than something flashy. Less is more. November happens to be epilepsy awareness month, so I looked for tattoo artists in my area and found one in Jersey City hoping to set up a date in November.

It was nerve-racking going alone into a tattoo parlor no less, but I went in and described what I wanted, a geometric brain showing the right hemisphere. I also wanted the right temporal lobe colored purple. The artist told me she'd work on it, and I scheduled a date for a couple of days later.

On November 7th, 2016, I headed to the tattoo shop right after work. I checked in and looked at the design the artist had put together. I liked it but had her change one or two lines to separate the lobes of the brain and make things a little cleaner. Not long after checking in, I was in one of the chairs getting prepped. They put the stencil on my right forearm, and I looked in the mirror. It looked great to me. I gave the okay, and we began.

I honestly thought the process would hurt more. It somewhat felt like pulling a bandage off slowly and feeling the hairs it's attached to rip off as well. With that said, the needle wasn't too dreadfully painful. The whole process only lasted for about an hour. Before I knew it, the tattoo artist was done. I was both excited and happy about how it turned out.

A lot of people are intrigued when they see it, and the common question is, "Why is that part purple?" Most of the time, I say, "I suffer/used to suffer from seizures. That's the part of my brain where they originated. Also, the color for epilepsy awareness is purple."

My tattoo made me feel normal if at least for the day. Meanwhile, Dr. Kapoor kept weighing my options and introducing me to medical experts.

In December 2016, I learned about another type of surgery, which uses a laser to ablate seizure focuses thermally. After hearing about its potential success, I agreed to meet a representative of Monteris Medical named Jerry. We met at a Dunkin' Donuts to discuss what he could do.

He explained that Monteris Medical was a biotech company that developed MRI-guided thermal ablation technology. Jerry said their Robotic Surgical Assistant (ROSA) could perform a specialized type of procedure called laser ablation. I would first receive a Stereo EEG (SEEG), which would have the neurosurgeon implant electrodes into my brain. After having seizures, the focus could be found with great accuracy. An SEEG seemed leaps and bounds more accurate than a regular EEG. After finding the focus of my seizures, I could receive a second surgery, the corrective one, if the seizure focus was safe for removal. This is where laser ablation came in.

This surgery would use ROSA once again, and the doctor would locate the focus found during the SEEG and use heat to burn out, or ablate, the affected brain tissue. In theory, it would rid me of my seizures. Jerry was very professional and answered every question I had from the surgery specifics to healing time. The healing time was not long at all. This surgery option was as minimally invasive as it gets. Before our meeting, I only knew about corrective surgeries, which would leave you with a massive scar on either side of your head. This surgery would leave minimal scarring.

With all the good things like the minimal invasiveness aside, it did seem rather risky. My mother, who was with me, was wary, but I knew it was my decision and felt this was the route to go.

I trusted Jerry and scheduled an appointment in New York City with Dr. Saadi Ghatan, a well-respected neurosurgeon, in the fourth quarter of 2016. Luckily, at the time, I'd worked as a secretary in a mental health office at a hospital in Jersey City, and my health insurance made it possible to see such reputable doctors. Dr. Ghatan specialized in pediatric neurosurgery, and that was a plus. If he could work on small child-sized brains, working on an adult brain could be easier for him in theory.

I'd met Dr. Ghatan for the first time with my mother. He explained my options if corrective surgery was not viable via laser ablation. One option was vagus nerve stimulation (VNS). The vagus nerve starts in the brain and runs down the spine and is responsible for a lot of involuntary body functions, like heartbeat and digestive tract.

Dr. Ghatan said, "This is not a cure, but rather a way to cope with your disorder that entails placing a magnet in the chest, which is connected to a device (stimulator) in the brain via the vagus nerve. Then a special bracelet is worn, which interacts with the magnet in the chest to send an electric impulse to the seizure focus area and curbs any seizure activity."

It wasn't a viable option at the time due to the lack of knowledge we had of my seizures, but it would be good to familiarize myself with some potential procedures, which could help me. If nothing else was able to help me, this could be a good option for me because my auras gave me a heads up when a seizure was occurring. I'd be able to touch the bracelet to my chest and hopefully stop a seizure from occurring.

I was worried, but during our visit, I found myself believing in Dr. Ghatan's faith in me. He told me right then, "Look at this picture. I wouldn't recommend doing anything to you that I wouldn't do to my own children."

That sentence alone made me respect him. There might be doctors who would risk someone's well-being to try a surgery that may not work, but he seemed so honest and confident in himself. He also worked closely with Dr. Lara Marcuse, a neurologist.

I felt bad that I was phasing Dr. Kapoor out of my life and not seeing him felt wrong. However, at that point, the doctors who could help me, even more, were in New York City, and I needed to commit to them entirely.

By that time, my seizures seemed to be coming fast and furious. I had a monster seizure on November 29th, and then in December, I had six more spread across the month.

I was concerned and miserable about my situation. Something had to be done quickly.

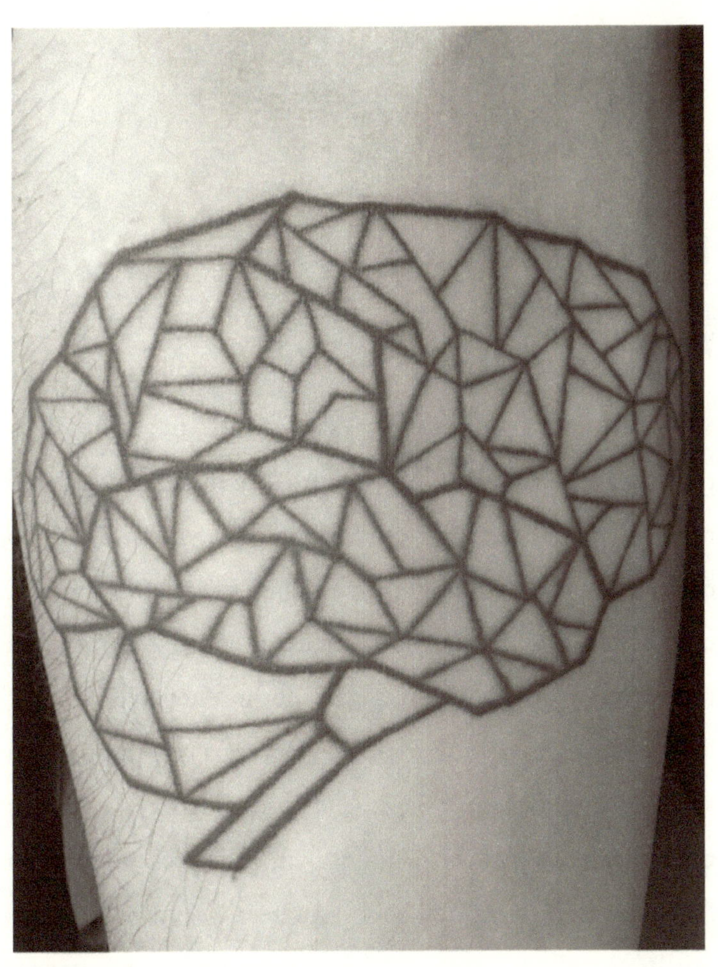

My first tattoo.

15

WADA

Although I would've loved to jump into having surgery and rid myself of my seizures, that would've been
medical malpractice. Since I had new doctors, I had to
do a lot of my old tests all over again for their records. I
had MRIs and EEGs as well as a neuropsychological
test. A neuropsych test is a very comprehensive psycho-
logical performance test that evaluates everything from
speech, memory and hand-eye coordination to assess
cognitive brain function. Due to my seizures originating
from my right temporal lobe, this test would help figure
out how well my temporal lobes were working concerning memory and speech.

The length of the test felt like a marathon. When
one task was over, a new one would start. There was a
portion where I had to repeat words spoken to me. I had
to remember a certain word, which the doctor would ask

me to repeat about an hour later, and I had to repeat a list of numbers said to me in descending order, then another list in ascending order.

One of my favorite parts was having a story read to me and having to repeat it back by giving the most important plot points. There was also a tactile portion of the test where I had to insert pegs into their respective holes in a certain amount of time.

I recall this test lasting anywhere from two to two and a half hours.

Things went well, but there were even more tests conducted to further assess my brain function. The next test could've been the most important one out of any I had taken, and I was scheduled at Mount Sinai Hospital in Uptown Manhattan in late May of 2017. It was called a Wada.

The objective of the test is to figure out which hemisphere of my brain was dominant. Since I'm right-handed, my left hemisphere should be dominant. A left-handed person would most usually have a dominant right hemisphere.

The idea here is to ascertain if it would be safe to operate on my right temporal lobe. If it turns out my right hemisphere is dominant, then VNS surgery might be the best option. However, if my left hemisphere was dominant, as expected, laser ablation could be the best way to go.

I remember the day of the procedure. Lou and I woke up early, around 4:30 a.m. because check-in at the hospital was relatively early. We left our apartment at around 5 a.m. and got into the city quickly. Before we knew it, we were at Mount Sinai Hospital. I checked in at the security desk and told them I had a procedure scheduled. They directed me to registration where all my insurance and financial formalities were sorted out.

Then I made my way to the neurology department. When I got to the correct floor, it was eerily quiet. I had never been there so early in the day. A lot of lights were off. I had found a note on one of the walls that told me where to go, and I finally met the technician who would be setting up my EEG for the Wada.

I followed her to the application room and took a seat in a comfortable chair. I've stated it before, EEG application can be quite relaxing, but pair it with the fact that the EEG tech was playing Enya in the background, the hospital felt like it had turned into a spa. I'm surprised I was able to stay awake. It was so early and relaxing. Lou fell asleep in the waiting room.

After all the electrodes were applied and my head was wrapped up, I was ready for the Wada. The technician took me downstairs where I had to undress and change into a hospital gown. Then I was taken to the room where one of the most jarring experiences of my life would take place.

There were monitors all over the room plus a gurney-style bed and a huge window with some onlookers. Some of my doctors would be witnessing my Wada. It comforted me to know that they were there. I felt like they had everything under control.

One of the biggest risks of doing Wada is the possibility of a stroke. You're probably wondering why a stroke might occur. Don't worry. I'll explain what occurs during this procedure in detail.

I lay on the gurney, answered a series of questions, and got prepped. The first step would be inserting a needle into my femoral artery in my groin. Knowing this before the procedure didn't bother me too much, but while I lay there, realizing it was about to happen, I started to freak out a bit.

My hospital gown got removed, and I lay there exposed in front of the doctors and staff. The uneasiness I felt from this was strong. Sterile drapes were placed on top of me to cover the areas the doctors didn't need access to, like my chest and lower legs. The room was freezing, but thankfully the bed had the ability to warm itself up.

The medical staff rubbed my groin area with an alcohol pad and then proceeded to insert the needle. They said I'd feel some burning as the numbing agent was administered. That was an understatement. I winced but tried to stay as still as possible. The combination of the needle and the burning in such a sensitive area made things quite uncomfortable. I was told to remain as still as possible, and the requests evolved from polite reminders to strict orders. I don't blame them. I had a hard time getting over what was going on.

Little did I know that the first needle was only to apply the numbing agent. The real needle came next, and it went into my femoral artery and was swapped for a catheter once successfully in the artery. The pressure of the medical staff's fingers in the area made me think it was the needle poking around at the artery. It was a surreal experience. Although my groin area was numb, I was still able to feel the pressure, and I could hardly keep still as my mind made me overthink the situation.

Once the catheter took the place of the needle in the groin, it was extended into the carotid artery all the way into my neck. Yes, you read that right. The catheter extended about three feet through my femoral artery up to my neck. Luckily, I didn't feel any of it.

Next, while the catheter was in my carotid artery, the staff injected contrast to see the blood vessels supplying blood to different parts of my brain. After the contrast was administered, I felt a warm sensation over my face and developed a metallic taste in my mouth as they studied one half of my brain at a time.

After pictures were taken, the neurological testing started. Using the same blood vessel used to administer the contrast, medication was inserted to sedate one-half of my brain at a time.

I recall coming to and hyperventilating. The doctors surrounding me tried to calm me down, all while one-half of my brain was asleep. Once I did calm down, they started different tests.

I had to point to certain pictures that depicted a

word they said, and then the reverse was tried. I also re-call having to point to certain physical objects. The experience was dreamlike. At one point, I could barely point my finger at an item that corresponded to a word spoken to me.

When my brain's right hemisphere was asleep, I had to point with my right hand, and I could barely keep it straight. It swayed so much. Also, I was blind in my left eye. Each hemisphere controls the opposite side of the body. So, when my right hemisphere was sedated, I performed tasks with my right side and vice versa. The whole experience seemed out of this world. I was blind in both eyes at different points, and I still can't express in words how wild that experience was.

Another test involved repeating phrases and words so the doctors could ascertain which hemisphere played a major role in my speech and memory. When the sedative wore off and both hemispheres were conscious, I had to try to remember words and pictures shown to me from the previous round of sedation. I remember it being rather difficult. I remember having a slurred speech on both occasions, but one hemisphere edged out the other.

I couldn't tell you how long the procedure lasted since I was in and out of consciousness, but before I knew it, I was out of that cold room and in a hospital recovery bed. Lou met me there, and I asked him how many hours had passed. It was early afternoon, around 2 p.m.

I had to stay long enough to ensure I hadn't developed any blood clots, which could be a catalyst for a stroke, but about an hour later, I was able to go home. I had to take care not to disrupt my groin from healing. It would be sore for the next few days.

. . .

The Wada turned out to be a success! I spoke with the team in New York City, and the results inspired them. The tests confirmed my left hemisphere was dominant. So, Dr. Ghatan could use ROSA and an SEEG to find out exactly where my seizures were occurring. If this didn't end up leading to corrective surgery, we'd at least know where my seizures originated.

I was all for proceeding with the surgeries. However, I was a bit wary about it. Having electrodes hooked up to my brain was one thing but having parts of my brain burned out was another matter.

I'd spent time talking with my doctors, my mother and my brothers. I even spoke with some of my friends about my progress and far too often I was asked, "Can't you just live with seizures?" Sadly, not everyone knows how vicious seizures can actually be. Aside from the utter misery my seizures made me feel, every time they happened, there was a real threat of injury, or even death. After meeting countless medical professionals over the years, I learned about sudden unexpected death in epilepsy (SUDEP). SUDEP happens when a person who suffers from epilepsy suddenly dies without warning, with no other cause of death found. The thought of this scares me. The truly terrifying thing is how seizures can become more severe over time and you'll never know the severity of your next one until it's already happened. So yes, seizures can kill someone who suffers from epilepsy. Ultimately, it was my decision to go through with surgery and it seemed like the right one.

To prepare, I quit my sporadic smoking hobby cold turkey. I knew smoking leading up to any surgery was risky. I decided to be proactive and get to it months before my surgery in order to give my body a chance to get back to baseline. I wouldn't say it was hard because there was something much bigger in my future: life-changing surgery.

Obviously, I wanted it to go as well as medically possible. I also did some research on what to expect with both the SEEG and laser ablation surgeries. I'd be lying if I said pictures and video of the SEEG didn't worry me. One video showed a doctor drilling into a patient's skull so he could have access to the brain and implant the electrodes. The drilling part made me uneasy, but if there was a silver lining, at least I'd be under general anesthesia.

16

AUGUST SURGERY

2017 was filled with seizures. Some months, I only had one, but at other times, they came at me relentlessly every week. Some days, I had two or three. I even celebrated the Fourth of July by having a terrible seizure.

My SEEG was scheduled for August 4th with a tentative date for laser ablation surgery for August 18th, pending the findings of the SEEG. I led up to the August 4th surgery by having a double dose of seizures on the day of my 24th birthday on the 3rd.

I did my best to stay calm, but I was very worried. My emotions were all over the place. I had never had surgery before, and perhaps I was being biased, but brain surgery seemed way more daunting than surgery on an arm, leg, or some other part of the body.

When you take a second to think about it, your brain is you. Everything you know about yourself and anything else is because of your brain. If something went wrong, my whole being could be in real jeopardy.

I knew the temporal lobe, in the simplest description, deals with memory and emotions. I worried about my memory and emotions following a surgery that would get rid of part of my temporal lobe. I worried about whether I would still be the same person.

In other words, would I still like the things I enjoyed, like baseball, music and movies? There is also a paradox that still sticks with me and freaks me out when I think of it. The fact that the temporal lobe deals with memory and a portion of mine was being removed, I could have forgotten something as a result but not know I forgot it because I wouldn't remember it in the first place. Yikes.

My pre-op appointments were pretty generic. My weight, height and other vitals were checked, and I had blood drawn. They focused on whether or not anesthesia had been a problem for me in the past. I had never had surgery before, so I could not answer definitively. As far as I knew, I didn't have an allergy to anesthesia.

On the 2nd of August, I had two seizures, one before work and one during my lunch break in a nearby park.

Jeez. Still, my coworkers made me feel appreciated and got me gifts. I took my birthday off from work so I could relax. My birthday also started about a month of medical leave granted to me so I could have time off for these surgeries.

I went to Max Brenner, a restaurant in New York City for a birthday dinner, and meandered the city a bit, but I was in a bit of a fog. When I got home, all I could think of was the upcoming surgery.

It didn't help that I stayed up till past midnight and then couldn't sleep. I listened to music and, being a sports fan, read some of Joe Buck's autobiography, all the while knowing I had to leave at 4:10 a.m. to arrive at Mount Sinai West by 5:30 a.m. By the time I took an Uber and got to New York City via the Lincoln Tunnel, I was exhausted.

My head cleared after I checked in at Mount Sinai West because they keep the place so cold. It was the dead of summer outside, so I had shorts on. It was freezing inside.

The nurses checked my vitals and then applied an IV. Soon after, my mom showed up to help keep me calm. Right after that, Dr. Ghatan arrived to greet me and let me know everything would be okay. His presence made me feel somewhat calmer despite having the thought of having a dozen electrodes drilled through my skull and implanted in my brain. No wonder I couldn't sleep that morning.

When it was time to be taken to the surgery room, I said goodbye to my mother, and she wished me luck. I remember entering the surgery room and seeing ROSA in person for the first time. Next, I was having anesthesia applied, and then I was asleep.

I don't remember much after that, but my surgery was performed with ROSA by Dr. Ghatan without a hitch. I was lucky to have him on my team.

Waking up was great but scary. I knew right where I was, and my head was on fire. I was nauseous and had a terrible pain in my temples. I started hyperventilating and crying in what seemed like an involuntary rage. As hard as I tried not to be, I was mean to the nurses. I hadn't had so much as a drink of water in more than twelve hours, and I was no camel. I needed water.

I dozed off and woke up around 4:30 p.m. I felt a little better but was still dehydrated. I had apple juice and found out they had the YES network on the TV so I could watch the Yankees.

That idea didn't last long because I was so nauseous from the anesthesia's side effects. I felt a little better after I threw up several times. Still, my jaw ached because the doctor had drilled through several muscles necessary for chewing.

The bill of fare wasn't great. I got to slurp apple sauce and Jell-O, and that was about it. The scent of better meals, like pasta or burgers, had me reaching for the vomit bucket.

Periodically, the neurologists would stop by my room, check on me to ask how I was doing and check my memory by asking general knowledge questions, like who the president was. They didn't bother telling me how the Yankees were doing.

The following day, my head still hurt when I opened my mouth or bit down, so I'm sorry to say the Jell-O fest continued. Mostly, I lay in bed, bored.

Later, Dr. Marcuse came by and said she spotted a part of my brain that was abnormal. Hearing that the doctors were able to find something so quickly was reassuring. I was still off meds when my mom came to visit. It was late, and she looked tired. I probably looked fairly ghastly myself.

On the 6th, I could barely sleep but didn't have to worry about the pain in my jaw from chewing since I had no appetite. I pondered the worth of the surgeries and giving up. Nurses buzzed around like so many bees, and then they moved me to another room.

It took a while to set up my new monitor, and the whole time I was very nauseous. I texted Dr. Marcuse about how my nausea made me want to quit.

By that night, I'd had enough. I asked for pain meds for the pressure in my head, and while waiting, I had an aura and clicked the record button, which would tell the computer to timestamp the button press and allow my doctors to easily look back and observe my brain's electrical activity at that precise moment. Before I knew it, there were six to eight nurses in my room shouting things. I couldn't stay still. I was weak and delirious.

Nurses were shouting at me to remain lying down for my safety, but I was trying to sit up for some reason.

I was delirious and felt the most comfortable position would be sitting up. However, the nurses continued to hold me down, and I continued to try to shake them off. They must've thought I was still having the seizure.

A nurse exclaimed, "He's so strong!"

I was not relenting. Despite the staff of six to eight nurses attempting to hold me down, I was successful at not being subdued. I wasn't intentionally being difficult.

The time immediately following a seizure is called the postictal phase and is why I was so delirious and unable to follow the nurses' requests.

Afterward, I felt bad for my mother. From what I'd heard, she was hysterical. It was my first grand mal seizure, and it caught us both by surprise. She was worried about my safety, and luckily, I was in the hospital and safe once the seizure subsided.

Safe in the hospital or not, things weren't getting better. Having a grand mal seizure is frightening. It's the type of seizure most people think of when they hear about a seizure because it can be violent.

During a grand mal's tonic phase, you lose consciousness, and your muscles contract. If you are standing, you'll fall, which is dangerous. Many people are injured from the fall itself, usually because they strike their head on a table, a chair, or the floor.

After about twenty seconds, the clonic phase starts, and all your muscles start a rhythmic series of flexing and relaxing. The contractions can last for more than two minutes.

Without being dramatic, the seizure is scary for the patient and those who see it. The person enduring a seizure may mumble or scream as the seizure starts. Afterward, they are at the whims of a brain electrically stimulated strangely and frighteningly.

Confusion afterward is common, which may be present immediately after regaining consciousness and may last quite a while. Sometimes, a severe headache plagues the victim.

Later, I also had a normal—for me—complex partial seizure during the SEEG. Having my normal seizure made me feel a little better than just having the grand mal because it would show my doctor what normally happens to me.

The next morning, Dr. Marcuse told me that my two seizures were more than enough data. That meant the electrodes would get removed on the 8th. She told me she loved what she saw during the monitoring. She said the removal would take place in under an hour.

Before I went under, I asked the anesthesiologist the time and then told him I'm trying to make it back in time to catch the beginning of the Yankees game. He laughed. During all the drama, I've realized the little things, like baseball, were keeping me sane.

After the electrodes were removed from my brain/skull, I had twelve wounds that needed stitching and was soon able to be discharged. I worried incessantly about not scratching the stitches, which is a real testament to the technology used if my biggest fear was making sure I didn't scratch my stitches.

I had some neck pain the next day, perhaps from a pinched nerve suffered during my grand mal seizure, but otherwise, I was happy to get some fresh air.

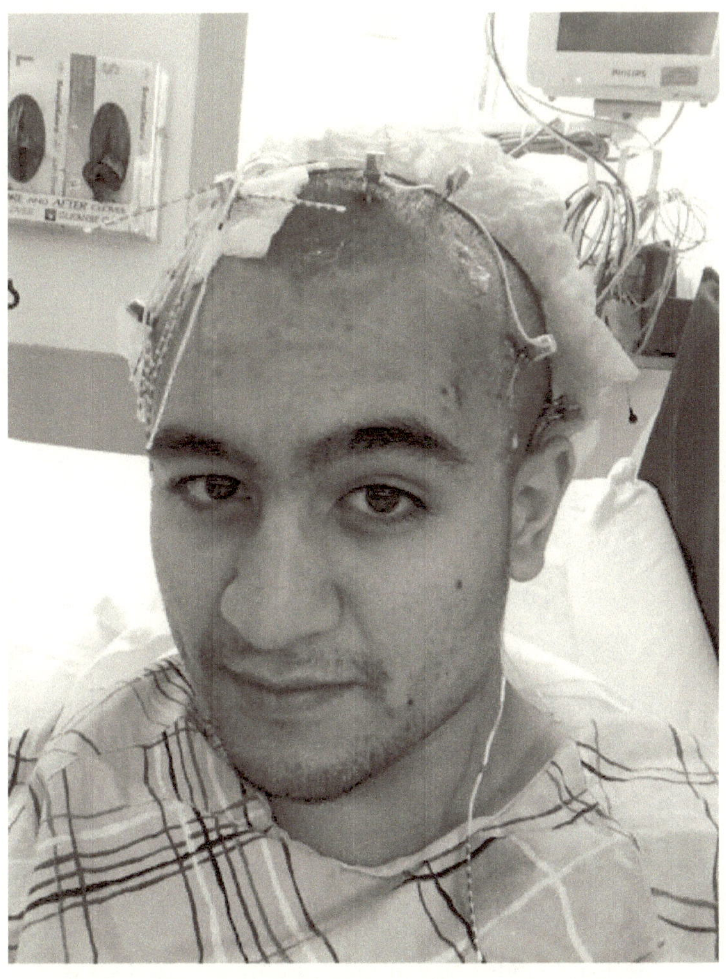

A picture of me before my electrode removal. You can see how the electrodes protruded out of my skull at different points.

17

HALFWAY

I was happy to have the first half of my surgeries out of the way, and I had friends and coworkers who checked up on me during the month I was in and out of the hospital. They showed compassion and were sympathetic.

The picture I took before my electrode removal is one of my favorite pictures of myself. It's one thing to tell the story but another thing to show pictures. People are often intrigued when I show them the picture while others get squeamish.

My boss at the mental health office I worked for at the time was all for me taking leave to take care of my health, and she wanted to know if I was doing well during my time off. She was always great, and I always appreciated her understanding.

I wasn't as nervous about the second surgery as I was for the first surgery, but I was for sure uneasy. I wanted to get to the hospital as quickly as possible and start the process. I would be losing a part of my brain, and once again, I was faced with the reality that if something went wrong, I could be completely changed forever. My doctors explained to me after the findings of my SEEG that my right hippocampus and amygdala were where my seizures originated. They were going to be removed, and I could only hope my doctor knew what he was doing.

Time seemed to be in slow motion the week and a half leading up to surgery, and I was thrilled to meet with Dr. Ghatan to go over surgery logistics on the 16th. I had multiple questions, but he was serene and assuring as always. Afterward, I had stopped at the Doughnut Project, an awesome doughnut spot in the city, to enjoy a couple of doughnuts and some normalcy.

18

THE OTHER HALF

On August 18th, my check-in and pre-op went much like my first surgery. I took an Uber to Mount Sinai West, and mom and Hector came along. I registered and pretty much remained quiet and kept to myself. Once again, I was beyond thirsty, but you can't drink anything due to surgery rules. I lay in my hospital bed, waiting for my life to be changed, hoping I would be well enough to watch the Yankees later.

Before I knew it, I was waking up after the corrective surgery. I realized I had no pants on, and a catheter inserted to help me urinate. I complained to the nurse that I had to use the bathroom, but I couldn't get over the mental hurdle of the catheter running up my urethra to my bladder.

After much complaining, a nurse decided to help me

out by removing the catheter. There was no countdown to get me ready, just a swift tug, which caught me by surprise. I thought I had been ripped open. The pain was brief. The ripping-off-a-bandage analogy works in this instance. However, don't let the brief pain fool you. It was intense and radiated throughout my body.

I guarantee you no man would want to go through that. I exclaimed a few expletives after the nurse tugged, which I apologized for a little while later. She understood and accepted my apology.

I celebrated the removal of the catheter by finally relieving myself into a plastic urinal. Later, for good measure, I threw up three times due to the anesthesia's side effects. Whoopie.

The corrective surgery left no pain. The hard part was waiting with the thought in the back of my mind that I could have a seizure at any moment. Having a seizure is like walking outside during a thunderstorm. You're trying to run for cover because at any moment you can be struck by lightning. But the cover is non-existent. A person living with epilepsy always feels like they'll never get to cover because seizures control their life. They sneak up on you and attack.

I was well enough to be discharged the next day, but for some reason, my insurance company wouldn't approve my medication although I'd been on it for a while. So, I sat in my room and waited for an MRI with contrast. Afterward, I had some chicken soup, happy that my jaw didn't ache as it had after my first surgery.

On August 20th, I was discharged around 1 p.m. The insurance issue got straightened out, and I got my two prescriptions and headed home. I looked forward to having a shower and lying down.

Late summer in 2018, the upcoming solar eclipse gripped most of the world. Protective glasses were being sold, given out for free and even bundled with food orders by some restaurants. I don't understand how someone could trust shoddily constructed glasses to look directly at the blazing sun, but I had other things to worry about. I worried about recovering from brain surgery and staying seizure-free. Somehow health issues put things into perspective.

I was drowsy and slept a lot the next few days, but I was looking forward to seeing the Yankees live on the 25th. That was pretty amazing. Corrective brain surgery a week ago, and I was already heading out to Yankee Stadium. Still, I felt as if I was at risk of having a seizure at any time - exciting and scary at the same time.

The baseball game was exciting. The Yanks played great, but the Mariners took the game 2-1 in extra innings. It happens.

I had developed slight tinnitus in my ear - the loud crowd probably didn't help - but got cleared by Dr. Marcuse to return to work in mid-September. That was the easy part.

The tough part was waiting three hours at employee health for a more specific clearance letter that needed to list any explicit restrictions for my return to work. The only restriction I had was not lifting more than ten pounds. When I did get back to work, there was the usual chaos. It was like I had never left.

There were lots of well-wishers, checking up on me and asking how I was doing. It was nice but still stressful to be back and I still worried about having a seizure.

The thing is, I couldn't feel better yet. I had to wait to see whether or not seizures would continue to plague me. It was a waiting game. By the time I returned to work, I had gone a month seizure-free. I knew that something good was happening, but there was still worry about my epilepsy status. However, I was excited about my progress. Going a month seizure-free was something I would never have envisioned myself being able to achieve without my doctors and the surgeries.

On the bright side, I had very minimal scarring. I like to keep my hair short, and I have small scars on my scalp. However, you probably wouldn't notice them if you weren't looking for them. Once again, after going through two major brain surgeries, the minor scars are a testament to the technology Monteris provides.

19

SEIZURE-FREE BUT CAUTIOUS

No matter what, there's still a nagging feeling creeping up in my thoughts that I could have a seizure at any time. Although I was doing well, it was and still is difficult to shake the grasp seizures had on me.

I got to see Dr. Kapoor at the end of September to update him on my progress. He seemed very pleased with my recovery and, as always, was warm and supportive.

The next month, I'd returned to Mount Sinai and was cleared of any physical limitations. It was great news because I'd been thinking about registering for the epilepsy 5K run in Jersey City at the end of October, and now I could. Still, when I went home and tried to take care of some bills, I ran into roadblocks. Strange charges, unanswered phones and the bills were all ridiculous amounts!

It was great getting my life back, but sometimes everything seemed like an obstacle. On the day of the run, I headed out to Doughnut Project and took the PATH train to New York City. As any New Yorker knows, the MTA or PATH train service can be jerky when standing on the moving train. At some point during the trip, the brakes got pressed a bit too abruptly, and my head hit one of the vertical hand poles that was right beside me. I'm anxious by nature, and with the head bump being so close to my surgeries, I thought maybe I hurt my brain somehow.

It was scary, going to the city and proceeding like my day was normal. I realized I was okay as time passed and figured I was just paranoid. If you ever have brain surgery where your skull gets drilled in a dozen different points, you might not want to bang your head.

Later on, I ran the 5K and finished 11th. That was good, but I was disappointed that there were so few runners since I knew the Earth Day 5K that same year had over 360. Epilepsy is still an obscure disorder that many people seem to ignore.

The next month, while leaving my apartment to

head to work, I neglected to notice the frozen stairs which must've been wet by rain overnight. I took the status of the stairs for granted and swiftly began to descend them.

My feet flew out from under me, and I landed on one of the stairs on my behind. My lower back hit the stair above the one I landed on, and the abrupt stop of the fall had a slight whiplash effect on me. The jarring shake to my head scared me, and I became a little paranoid.

My hospital job made it so I could excuse myself and head to the ER. After a brief wait, I was seen and taken to get a CT scan. The doctor talked to me and said everything seemed normal. However, he did ask if I knew I had a rather small right hippocampus. I laughed and told him about my laser ablation surgery to thermally ablate my right hippocampus to destroy my seizure focus. He thought it was rather intriguing. I was discharged and I headed back to work. The fall hadn't done any harm.

Still, after my surgeries, people had a hard time empathizing with me about forgetting things.

My short-term memory sometimes isn't the best,

and that would make sense based on the parts of my brain that were removed. I guess people have a hard time grasping the fact that my brain was altered permanently.

Over the next couple of months, I got back into the grind of working daily, and things seemed back to normal. Then I got a call from Jerry at Monteris Medical.

20

MINNESOTA NICE

The year 2018 was a joy to behold. I was seizure-free for over four months and heading to Minnesota.

In December 2017, Jerry from Monteris Medical called to give me a heads up that Monteris Medical was interested in my story. He told me to expect a call from a representative, who might want to invite me to an event in Minnesota. I was elated. His call made a monotonous day at work seem awesome.

Not too long after Jerry's call, a woman named Samantha from Monteris called with information about what exactly she had planned. She seemed really nice and genuinely excited about this opportunity for me. She told me it would be a holiday work party taking place in January. She also told me a lot of Monteris employees, as well as the CEO, would be there to hear my story. I accepted the opportunity. Samantha told me she would email me all the logistics regarding flight and hotel info.

A few days later, I had met with Jerry to work on a promotional video for the meeting. We filmed in the lobby of a hotel where he asked me some questions about my surgery and got some B-roll shots to put together a nice video package.

I took a flight on the 26th that finally took off after being delayed twice, most likely due to weather, which made me a bit nervous, but the ride was smooth and uneventful. Lou was gracious enough to accompany me on my trip. I appreciated him for doing that because it was nice having someone with me. Lou fell asleep on the plane, but I couldn't. Instead of sleeping, I listened to the radio and a lot of music to pass the time on the roughly three-hour flight.

Upon arriving, we took a car to our hotel, and the driver's name was Joe, too. I thought that was pretty cool. He asked if I was in Minneapolis for business or pleasure. I told him business, and I felt like a VIP saying that.

At the hotel, we met Samantha, who gave me a gift bag with a Super Bowl shirt since the game was on that coming Sunday in Minneapolis. They gave me the event arrival time, and Lou and I had some extra time to explore the nearby surroundings. We walked around and saw some of the events for the Super Bowl. We didn't have a ton of time but were able to see some pretty fun stuff. I noticed a lot of strangers greet you in Minnesota. People from New York City and the surrounding area can sometimes get a reputation for being rude. I did not get that impression from the people of Minnesota. I found myself saying hi to strangers during our walk around the hotel area.

The beginning of the trip was great. It culminated with me taking the stage and doing an interview in front of a large crowd of Monteris employees. I was a lot more comfortable than I thought I'd be. I talked like I had done these dozens of times before. I made the crowd laugh with my hospital catheter story and the "He's so strong" part, too. It was a good time.

I started to tear up at the end of the interview when I realized this might all be behind me. The event helped me come to that reality. Afterward, people kept coming up to me to thank me for coming and making a difference. There was one employee who asked me how I liked Minnesota. I told him it was nice, and everyone seemed hospitable. He proceeded to tell me about a thing called "Minnesota nice." That's a stereotypical behavior people from Minnesota exhibit. It even has a Wikipedia page! It now made sense why complete strangers were so courteous.

The Monteris reps gave me an open tab, but I only had a burger after the speech in the hotel restaurant. When they found out that's all I had eaten, they gave me such a hard time!

The trip signified my first time on a flight, and it was great as Minnesota was great. I only wish I could've stayed longer.

21

THE DMV

I can't say I've ever heard about the DMV being compassionate, but right about April Fools' Day in 2018, I'd received a letter from the DMV stating I was cleared to drive if I agreed to keep them informed of my seizure status every six months for the next two years.

It might not seem like a big deal to some people, but when I obtained my license letter, I was elated. It was a small victory. I took a picture of the part, which told me I was eligible to get my license restored and posted it to my Instagram page.

I received supportive messages from people who were happy for me. That was great. When I had my license before my suspension, I didn't really drive. I live in such an urban setting, so it's easier to use mass transit or walk. Finding a parking space where I live is like winning the lottery. It's not easy. Losing my license stung, but I didn't lose independence because of it. However, getting it back was a victory in itself because it proved to me that my seizures were behind me, and I say that in all humility because I know how sneaky seizures can be. Sure, as I'm writing this, I haven't had one in three and a half years, but I'm always worried about them. That worry will never go away.

22

NATIONAL WALK FOR EPILEPSY

I first heard about the National Walk for Epilepsy in 2018 on Instagram. I found it because I follow the Epilepsy Foundation's account, but I found out too late and missed it.

So, I had planned to attend the next one. I talked to my younger brother, D, about a potential trip to Washington, D.C., in April 2019 for the walk. He was pretty open to the idea. D likes to travel and had gone to D.C. before to photograph a sports event while he was a part of his college's newspaper. I figured he'd love to go back for another event and take some more pictures; he loves taking pictures.

Being a baseball fan, I also planned on seeing the Washington Nationals play while we were there. You know I'm a diehard Yankees fan, but ultimately, I'm a baseball fan. If I get the chance to see a game at an away stadium, I want to make it happen. So, D and I started planning.

We planned to head to D.C. on April 26th, 2019, when we could catch a Nationals game that night. The walk was the next day. We figured we would head back home later that day.

In the morning, D and I met in New York City to catch the bus that'd take us to D.C. We were set to leave at 7 a.m. and arrive around 11 a.m., so we stopped for some coffee and then boarded our bus. The ride wasn't as daunting as I'd expected it to be. Every time I checked the map on my phone, I was taken aback by how far we had traveled. Before I knew it, we had traveled through New Jersey and were in Maryland, then D.C.

Our drop-off spot was close to the White House, so it was the first landmark we stopped at after arriving in D.C. We walked around a lot and noticed scooters littering the sidewalks. We later found out that these were electric scooters for rent. You pay by the minute, but it's a fun and quick way to get around the city. Before we knew it, we were closing in on the Lincoln Memorial and admiring its grandiosity.

Shortly after arriving at the Lincoln Memorial, it started raining, and not just a few drops here and there. It was raining cats and dogs. Everyone huddled together for shelter under the Lincoln Memorial structure. D and I were worried the baseball game would be canceled, and I constantly checked for news regarding a delay or cancelation.

The rain was so bad that we decided to catch an Uber to get to our hotel to check in. Standing around and waiting for the rain to stop was a waste of time. Our hotel was in Arlington, Virginia, not too far away, and after checking in, we found our room had an awesome balcony. However, it was getting soaked, just like my sneakers, and I was worried they wouldn't dry for the walk the following morning.

The rain subsided, and we decided to kill some time by walking around to see what Virginia had to offer. I kept my eye on the news regarding the baseball game. Not canceled yet. Ultimately, we attended the game and had fun. We had cheesesteaks at the stadium and left a little early, so we'd be sure to get enough sleep to be ready for the walk the next morning.

My sneakers were still damp from the rain the afternoon before, but the weather on this Saturday morning was beautiful. Clear blue skies and not a cloud to be seen.

We checked in at the National Mall and got our event shirts. Then we got breakfast items, like bananas and granola bars, and looked at the booths with information about epilepsy, treatment methods, medications and such.

The walk was a 5K or just over three miles. It looped all around and gave participants a good chance to see various landmarks. I had fun walking with my brother, enjoying the landmarks and our conversations. At the end of the walk, D took lots of pictures of me, and we checked out more booths.

There was one booth giving free caricature drawings that looked like fun, so we stopped there, and each got one done. D.C. was extremely fun, and if it weren't for the coronavirus outbreak of 2020, which caused the 2020 National Walk for Epilepsy to become a virtual walk, D and I would have attended again.

The whole trip was a blast, and it helped me again feel comfortable in my skin and thankful I am seizure-free. I'm lucky.

I still take pride in my tattoo choice. Some of the best conversations I have had with others are the ones where they ask about my tattoo, or I show them a picture from one of my surgeries. It's funny to see their reaction when they see the electrodes sticking out of my head. Seeing it at first can be quite jarring.

I don't shy away from conversations about my ordeal. I love telling my story, but I like to spread the word and let others know about how great medical technology can be.

I often feel liberated, but I still worry about having another seizure. I don't think the fear of having another seizure will ever leave, but I am, without a doubt, grateful for every day that goes by where I stay seizure-free. I like to look toward the bright side. I am currently on only one medication. I remain on Vimpat just to be cautious, and hopefully one day, I can finally be medication-free.

Through it all, the seizures, the surgeries, and the worry and stress, I recall my mother telling my neurosurgeon, Dr. Ghatan, during a pre-surgery visit, "I'm worried my boy won't be the same."

To that worry, Dr. Ghatan assured her that I was in

good hands. I believed it. From the moment I'd met Dr. Ghatan, I knew he was right for me. He carried himself in such a confident and caring manner from the very beginning. I'm happy I had faith in him because he is one of the main reasons that I'm seizure-free today.

I really like that feeling.

www.ingramcontent.com/pod-product-compliance
Lightning Source LLC
Chambersburg PA
CBHW031345060726
47590CB00007B/2634